CW01210320

Urban Mastery:
Navigating Success in the Heart of the City

Josh Jones

Copyright Notice:

Copyright © 2024 by Josh Jones. All rights reserved. No part of this publication may be reproduced, distributed, or transmitted in any form or by any means, including photocopying, recording, or other electronic or mechanical methods, without the prior written permission of the publisher, except in the case of brief quotations embodied in critical reviews and certain other noncommercial uses permitted by copyright law.

Disclaimer:

This book is provided as is, without warranty of any kind, express or implied, including but not limited to the warranties of merchantability, fitness for a particular purpose, or non-infringement. The content is for informational purposes only and is not intended as professional advice. The use of this guide is solely at the reader's discretion. The author and publisher are not responsible for any actions taken by the reader based on the information provided herein.

"Heartbeat of the City"

In the city's heart, we find our beat, Among the bustling streets, our dreams we greet. Skyscrapers high, ambitions soar, In every corner, opportunity knocks on the door.

Lights that never fade, voices loud and clear, In the urban maze, we find our way, never fear. The city's rhythm, fast and bold, Tales of success, in these streets, are told.

A jungle of concrete, with a spirit free, Here, we discover who we're meant to be. In the heart of the city, our passions ignite, Under the urban stars, we find our light.

Embarking on a journey to thrive in the bustling environment of a big city requires more than just physical relocation; it necessitates a profound transformation of one's mindset. The urban landscape, with its relentless pace, towering skyscrapers, and mosaic of cultures, demands resilience, adaptability, and a proactive stance towards personal and professional challenges. To navigate this complex terrain successfully, one must cultivate what can aptly be termed the Urban Mindset—a psychological framework equipped to handle the unique pressures and opportunities that city life presents.

At the heart of developing an Urban Mindset is the concept of self-assessment. This process involves a candid evaluation of one's strengths and weaknesses, a task that is both challenging and essential. It requires introspection and honesty, as well as a willingness to accept feedback from others. Identifying your strengths allows you to leverage them more effectively, while acknowledging your weaknesses provides a roadmap for personal growth and development.

To begin, consider your resilience, a critical component of the Urban Mindset. Resilience is not just about enduring setbacks but also about bouncing back stronger. Ask yourself how you handle failure and stress. Do you see challenges as insurmountable obstacles, or do you view them as opportunities to learn and evolve? Cultivating resilience involves developing a positive outlook, practicing stress-reduction techniques, and setting realistic goals.

Adaptability is another key facet of thriving in an urban environment. The city is in a constant state of flux, with new opportunities and challenges arising daily. Assess how well you adapt to change. Do you find it difficult to deviate from your plans, or are you able to pivot quickly in response to new information? Enhancing your adaptability involves staying informed about industry trends, being open to new experiences, and learning to manage uncertainty with grace.

Networking prowess is also essential in the urban jungle. The vast majority of opportunities in the city, from career advancements to social engagements, arise from connections. Reflect on your networking skills. Are you comfortable initiating conversations with strangers? Do you maintain your professional relationships? Improving your networking skills can be as simple as attending more social events, joining professional associations, and being genuinely interested in others.

Time management is a critical skill in the fast-paced urban environment, where the demands on your time can be overwhelming. Evaluate your time management skills. Are you able to prioritize tasks effectively? Do you find yourself constantly rushing from one commitment to another, or do you allocate time for relaxation and self-care? Enhancing your time management skills requires setting clear priorities, learning to say no, and making use of productivity tools and techniques.

Finally, consider your cultural competence. The city is a melting pot of cultures, and the ability to interact respectfully and effectively with people from diverse backgrounds is invaluable. Assess your level of cultural awareness and sensitivity. Do you make an effort to understand the cultural norms and values of others? Are you open to different perspectives? Developing cultural competence involves educating yourself about other cultures, being open-minded, and practicing empathy.

In cultivating the Urban Mindset, the process of self-assessment is ongoing. As you grow and evolve, so too will your strengths and weaknesses. The key is to approach this process with curiosity and an openness to change. By doing so, you equip yourself with the psychological tools needed to thrive in the concrete jungle, turning the challenges of city life into stepping stones for personal and professional success.

This transformation does not occur overnight. It requires dedication, effort, and, most importantly, a willingness to step outside your comfort zone. But the rewards—personal growth, professional success, and the unparalleled vibrancy of urban life—are well worth the effort. As you navigate the complexities of the city, let your Urban Mindset be your guide, leading you to opportunities and experiences beyond your wildest dreams.

Understanding the intricate web of city infrastructure is akin to learning a new language. It's a crucial step for anyone aiming to thrive in the urban landscape, where the ability to efficiently navigate transportation systems, secure appropriate housing, and utilise city services can significantly enhance one's quality of life. This chapter delves into the practicalities of city living, offering insights and strategies to demystify the urban maze and empower you to make the most of the opportunities and amenities at your disposal.

Transportation in the city is the lifeline that connects its diverse parts, making the mastery of its systems paramount. Public transport, often comprehensive in large cities, can be a reliable, cost-effective, and environmentally friendly option for getting around. Familiarise yourself with the local transit network, which may include buses, trams, undergrounds, and trains. Many cities offer dedicated apps or websites that provide real-time updates, route planners, and ticketing options, making it easier to plan your journey efficiently. Consider purchasing season tickets or travel cards if you're a frequent traveller, as these can offer considerable savings.

For those occasions when public transport doesn't suit your needs, explore alternative modes of transportation. Cycling is not only healthy but also allows you to bypass traffic congestion. Many cities have invested in cycling infrastructure, such as dedicated bike lanes and bike-sharing schemes, to facilitate this mode of transport. Additionally, ride-sharing apps and taxi services can offer convenience for those out-of-reach destinations or when time is of the essence. Remember, the key to mastering urban transportation lies in understanding the options available and selecting the most suitable one based on your destination, time, and budget.

Housing in the city presents its own set of challenges and opportunities. The search for a place to call home requires a balance between affordability, location, and suitability. Start by defining your priorities, such as proximity to work or educational institutions, access to public transport, and the availability of local amenities like shops, parks, and leisure facilities. Be prepared to compromise, as finding the perfect place within your budget can be competitive in popular urban areas.

Engage in thorough research to understand the nuances of the city's housing market. Online property portals, local newspapers, and real estate agents can provide valuable insights into available properties and price ranges. Consider the merits of different types of accommodation, from apartments and flats to shared houses, each with its own advantages and considerations. Security deposits, rental agreements, and utility bills are critical factors to understand before making a commitment.

City services encompass a wide range of public amenities and resources designed to improve residents' lives. Familiarising yourself with these services can significantly enhance your urban living experience. Libraries, community centres, and parks offer recreational and educational opportunities, often at little or no cost. Waste and recycling services are essential for maintaining a clean and sustainable living environment, so make sure to understand the local regulations and schedules.

Healthcare and emergency services are fundamental aspects of city infrastructure. Know how to access medical facilities, register with a local doctor, and what to do in an emergency. Additionally, staying informed about local government services and initiatives can provide access to support and resources in areas such as employment, education, and social services.

In conclusion, navigating the maze of city infrastructure requires a proactive approach and willingness to learn. By mastering the transportation network, making informed choices about housing, and utilising city services, you can significantly enhance your urban living experience. The city offers a dynamic and vibrant environment, and with the right knowledge and tools at your disposal, you can thrive in the heart of the urban jungle.

In the pulsating heart of the city, where ambitions soar as high as the skyscrapers and the streets are alive with a myriad of cultures and opportunities, the art of networking transforms into an essential skill for success. Building your urban tribe, a network of like-minded individuals who offer support, inspiration, and opportunities, is not merely about expanding your social circle; it's about creating a community that fuels your growth and amplifies your impact in the urban landscape.

The foundation of effective networking in such a bustling environment lies in recognising the value of genuine connections over mere acquaintances. This entails a shift from traditional networking views that often prioritise quantity over quality. The essence of building your urban tribe is to foster relationships based on shared interests, mutual respect, and a genuine interest in the success of others.

Initiating this journey requires a proactive stance. Begin by identifying your interests, both professional and personal, as these will guide you towards events, forums, and spaces where you can meet like-minded individuals. Whether it's a professional conference, a workshop, an art exhibition, or a community project, each event is a potential gateway to new connections. Embrace the diversity of the city by attending events that not only align with your existing interests but also expand your horizons to new fields and cultures.

Engaging in conversation with strangers can be daunting, yet mastering this skill is crucial for effective networking. Approach conversations with curiosity and an open mind, showing genuine interest in the other person's experiences, ideas, and aspirations. Remember, networking is a two-way street; it's as much about listening and learning as it is about sharing your own story. A helpful strategy is to prepare a set of open-ended questions that can help kickstart conversations and uncover common ground.

As you meet new people, focus on building a connection rather than immediately seeking favours or opportunities. Networking with the intention of giving rather than taking not only enriches the relationship but also sets a foundation of reciprocity and trust. Offer your skills, knowledge, or connections where they might benefit others, without an immediate expectation of return. This approach, often referred to as the principle of 'giving to get', lays the groundwork for a supportive and collaborative community.

In today's digital age, online platforms provide powerful tools for networking. Social media sites, professional networking platforms, and interest-based forums can help you connect with individuals and groups in your city and beyond. Use these platforms to share your insights, engage with others' content, and join conversations. However, digital connections should complement, not replace, face-to-face interactions. The most enduring relationships are often forged through personal interaction, where the nuances of body language and the energy of live conversations can create a deeper bond.

Follow-up is where many networking efforts falter. After making a connection, take the initiative to maintain the relationship. A simple message expressing your pleasure at meeting them, sharing an article relevant to your conversation, or suggesting a meet-up for coffee can keep the connection alive. Regular, meaningful interactions help transform initial acquaintances into a supportive network.

Remember, building your urban tribe is an ongoing process. Your network will evolve as you progress through different stages of your life and career. Some connections will naturally fade, while others will grow stronger and become integral to your journey. The key is to nurture your network with the same care and intention that you apply to your personal and professional development.

In essence, networking in the city is an art that blends strategy with authenticity. By approaching it with the right mindset and employing these strategies, you can build a vibrant urban tribe that supports your aspirations, enriches your life, and opens doors to new possibilities. The strength of your network lies not just in the numbers, but in the quality of connections and the shared journey towards success.

In the competitive city landscape, where opportunities come and go as swiftly as the passing metro, career acceleration becomes a pursuit not just of ambition, but of necessity. The urban professional environment is dynamic, demanding, and densely populated with talented individuals all vying for their chance to shine. To navigate this fast lane and not just survive but thrive, one must adopt a strategic approach, keenly aware of both the external opportunities and their internal compass of strengths and weaknesses.

The first step in this strategic approach is self-assessment, a critical exercise that serves as the foundation for personal and professional development. Identifying your strengths allows you to capitalise on them, turning what you're already good at into your greatest advantages. Conversely, recognising your weaknesses is not an admission of failure but a roadmap for growth, indicating where your efforts to improve could have the most significant impact.

Techniques for this self-assessment vary but often include reflection on past feedback, both positive and negative, from peers, supervisors, and mentors. Reflect on instances of success and failure alike; these are valuable indicators of where your natural talents lie and where there might be room for improvement. Personality tests and skills assessments can also offer insights, though they should not be taken as gospel but rather as additional data points to inform your understanding of yourself.

Armed with a clear picture of your strengths and weaknesses, the next step is to set targeted, achievable goals. These should be specific, measurable, attainable, relevant, and time-bound (SMART). For instance, if a recognised weakness is public speaking, a goal might be to attend a public speaking workshop and deliver a presentation within the next three months. Goals should play to your strengths too; if you excel at analytical thinking, seek opportunities that allow this skill to shine, such as leading a project that requires detailed data analysis.

Career acceleration in the city also requires a proactive stance on networking. Building a robust professional network is invaluable, offering insights into industry trends, upcoming opportunities, and advice from those who have navigated similar paths. Networking should not be reserved for formal events but integrated into your daily professional life. Engage with colleagues, join professional bodies relevant to your field, and don't shy away from reaching out to individuals whose career paths you admire. Remember, networking is about building genuine connections, not just collecting contacts.

Mentorship is another critical element. A mentor who has successfully navigated the urban professional landscape can offer guidance, support, and accountability. They can help you navigate your career path, offering advice on crucial decisions and introducing you to their network. Don't limit yourself to one mentor; different mentors can offer diverse perspectives and advice tailored to various aspects of your career and personal development.

Continuous learning is essential in a city that never stands still. Technologies evolve, industry trends shift, and new skills become crucial overnight. Stay ahead by committing to lifelong learning, whether through formal education, online courses, workshops, or self-study. Align your learning with your career goals, focusing on areas that will both address your weaknesses and bolster your strengths.

Finally, visibility is key in a competitive landscape. Make your achievements known in a manner that is professional and authentic. This can involve sharing successes in team meetings, contributing to company newsletters, or presenting at industry conferences.

Visibility ensures that when opportunities arise, your name is at the forefront of decision-makers' minds.

Career acceleration in the urban environment is not a linear journey; it's a complex navigation of personal development, strategic networking, continuous learning, and visibility. By understanding your own abilities and areas for improvement, and by strategically seizing the opportunities that the city offers, you can drive your career forward at pace, turning the competitive city landscape into a canvas of endless possibility.

Living in an urban environment presents unique financial challenges and opportunities. The pace of life, the cost of living, and the myriad ways to spend money can seem overwhelming. However, with the right approach, managing your finances in the city can not only be manageable but also incredibly rewarding, setting the stage for long-term financial security and prosperity. Developing financial savvy in the city requires a multifaceted approach, encompassing budgeting, saving, investing, and smart spending.

Budgeting is the cornerstone of effective financial management. It involves tracking your income and expenses to understand where your money goes each month. Start by listing your income sources, including wages, bonuses, and any other earnings. Next, categorise your expenses, starting with essentials like rent, utilities, groceries, and transport. Then, account for discretionary spending such as dining out, entertainment, and shopping. This exercise will highlight areas where you might overspend and where you can cut back. Budgeting apps and tools can simplify this process, offering insights into your spending habits and helping you stay on track.

Saving is crucial, especially in an expensive urban setting where unexpected expenses can arise suddenly. Aim to build an emergency fund covering at least three to six months of living expenses. This fund can be a financial lifeline in case of job loss, illness, or unforeseen expenses. Automating your savings can ensure you consistently set money aside before you have the chance to spend it. Direct a portion of your income into a separate savings account as soon as you receive your paycheck.

Investing is the next step towards financial growth. While it may seem daunting, investing is essential for building wealth over time, especially in an environment where the cost of living outpaces savings account interest rates. Start small, perhaps with a low-cost index fund or a robo-advisor, which can provide a diversified portfolio with minimal effort on your part. Educate yourself on the basics of investing, understanding risk, and the importance of a long-term perspective. Remember, investing involves risk, but not investing carries the risk of eroding your purchasing power over time due to inflation.

Smart spending in the city is about

making informed choices. Take advantage of the competitive urban market to find deals and discounts. Whether it's shopping for groceries, choosing a mobile plan, or subscribing to services, always look for value. Be mindful of lifestyle inflation, where increased income leads to increased spending on non-essential items. Instead, prioritise spending on experiences and purchases that genuinely add value to your life.

Additionally, consider side hustles or freelance work to boost your income. The gig economy is vibrant in urban settings, offering opportunities to earn extra money in flexible and creative ways. This additional income can accelerate your savings and investment goals.

Managing debt wisely is also crucial.

High-interest debt, such as credit card debt, can quickly undermine your financial health. Prioritise paying off high-interest debts and consider consolidating debts or negotiating lower interest rates where possible.

Finally, financial savvy includes planning for the future. This means not only saving for retirement but also considering insurance to protect against unforeseen events. Many urban professionals overlook the importance of health, disability, and life insurance, yet these can be crucial in protecting your financial future.

In conclusion, financial management in an urban setting requires diligence, education, and a proactive approach. By mastering the art of budgeting, saving, investing, and smart spending, you can navigate the financial challenges of city life and lay the foundation for a prosperous future. Remember, financial savvy is not innate; it's developed through practice, patience, and persistence.

In the heart of the bustling metropolis, amidst the concrete jungle and the cacophony of urban life, lies the oasis of tranquillity and rejuvenation – the city's green spaces. These pockets of nature, ranging from sprawling parks to hidden gardens, are not merely aesthetic enhancements but vital components for urban wellness. They offer a sanctuary for the soul, a place where one can reconnect with nature, breathe fresh air, and momentarily escape the relentless pace of city life. For those seeking balance and wellbeing in the urban environment, discovering and making the most of these green spaces becomes an essential pursuit.

The benefits of spending time in nature are well-documented, with research highlighting improvements in mental health, physical wellbeing, and cognitive function. In the urban context, where stress and sensory overload are commonplace, green spaces provide a crucial counterbalance. They offer a setting for relaxation and meditation, opportunities for physical activity, and a space for social interaction, all of which contribute to overall health and happiness.

To integrate these natural havens into your urban life, start by exploring the green spaces available in your city. Most metropolises boast a variety of parks, from the grand and historic to the small and community-focused. Each has its unique character and offerings, from wooded trails and water bodies to sports facilities and cultural events. Make it a mission to discover these areas, using city guides, apps, and websites dedicated to urban greenery. Make a list of spots to visit, and gradually tick them off as you explore each one.

Incorporating visits to these green spaces into your routine can be transformative. Start small by dedicating time each week to immerse yourself in these natural settings. Whether it's a morning jog in the park, a lunchtime stroll through a garden, or a weekend picnic with friends or family, regular engagement with nature can significantly enhance your quality of life. For those with a hectic schedule, even a brief respite in a green space can be revitalising. Find a bench where you can sit for a few moments, observe the natural beauty around you, and take deep, mindful breaths. This simple practice can help reduce stress and increase your sense of wellbeing.

Beyond passive enjoyment, actively engage with the natural environment to deepen your connection. This can include activities such as gardening in community plots, bird watching, or participating in conservation efforts. Many cities offer volunteer opportunities to help maintain and enhance their green spaces, providing a rewarding way to give back to the community while spending time outdoors.

Physical activity in green spaces is another key aspect of urban wellness. Parks often feature paths for walking, jogging, or cycling, as well as facilities for sports and exercise. These activities, set against the backdrop of nature, are not only beneficial for physical health but also more enjoyable and motivating than indoor workouts. Furthermore, engaging in physical activity outdoors provides exposure to natural light, which can help regulate sleep patterns and improve mood.

For those interested in mindfulness and meditation, green spaces offer the perfect setting. Practising mindfulness or meditating in a park can enhance the experience, allowing you to fully appreciate the sights, sounds, and smells of nature. This practice can help improve mental clarity, reduce stress, and promote a sense of peace and contentment.

Finally, urban green spaces are ideal for fostering community and social connections. They are gathering places where people from all walks of life come together, providing opportunities to meet new people, strengthen friendships, and participate in community events. This social aspect is integral to wellbeing, offering a sense of belonging and support.

In conclusion, the metropolis, with all its vibrancy and vitality, can also be a place of balance and wellbeing when we embrace its green spaces. By actively seeking out, appreciating, and utilising these natural havens, we can enhance our physical, mental, and social health. In the process, we not only enrich our own lives but also contribute to the wellbeing of the urban environment and its community.

Maintaining physical health in the urban milieu, with its fast-paced lifestyle, convenience food, and often sedentary jobs, presents a unique set of challenges. Yet, it is within this very environment that opportunities abound for those willing to embrace a proactive stance towards their health. The fit urbanite knows that staying healthy in the city is not merely about avoiding illness but about optimising well-being, energy levels, and physical fitness to thrive amidst the hustle and bustle.

Key to this urban wellness is the integration of regular physical activity into one's daily routine. The city landscape offers a variety of options to keep fit, from well-equipped gyms and fitness centres to public parks and greenways ideal for running, walking, or cycling. The trick is to find an activity that not only suits your fitness level and interests but also fits seamlessly into your schedule. This could mean opting for a gym that's close to your workplace or home, participating in fitness classes that coincide with your free time, or even incorporating exercise into your commute, such as cycling to work or getting off the bus a few stops early to walk the rest of the way.

Equally important is recognising the role of nutrition in maintaining physical health. The urban environment, with its plethora of dining out options and processed convenience foods, can make healthy eating seem like a daunting task. However, the informed urbanite sees the city's culinary diversity as an advantage. Farmers' markets, health food stores, and a wide array of restaurants offering healthy, nutritious meals are often at your doorstep. Planning your meals, cooking at home when possible, and making informed choices when dining out—opting for dishes rich in vegetables, lean proteins, and whole grains—can significantly contribute to your overall health.

Hydration is another cornerstone of physical well-being often overlooked in the urban rush. Carrying a reusable water bottle and opting for water or herbal teas instead of sugary drinks or excessive caffeine can improve hydration levels, aiding digestion, skin health, and energy levels.

The quality of sleep is paramount in the equation of urban health. The city's never-ending noise and lights can interfere with sleep patterns, making it essential to create a restful environment in your home. Strategies such as using blackout curtains, limiting screen time before bed, and establishing a calming pre-sleep routine can help improve the quality of your rest, thereby enhancing your physical and mental well-being.

Stress management is another crucial aspect of staying healthy in the city. The pressures of urban living can take a toll on one's physical health, making it essential to incorporate stress-reduction techniques into your lifestyle. This could include practices like yoga, meditation, deep-breathing exercises, or simply dedicating time to relax and enjoy leisure activities that bring you joy.

The urban environment also offers unique opportunities for staying active through unconventional means. Exploring the city on foot, participating in community sports leagues, or taking up new hobbies like dance classes or rock climbing can add variety to your fitness regimen, keeping you motivated and engaged.

Preventive health measures, such as regular check-ups and health screenings, are also part of the fit urbanite's toolkit. Taking advantage of the city's healthcare resources can help catch potential health issues early and keep you on track with your fitness goals.

In essence, staying healthy in the city requires a holistic approach that encompasses physical activity, nutrition, hydration, sleep, stress management, and preventive healthcare. By leveraging the unique resources and opportunities that urban living provides, you can navigate the challenges and embrace a lifestyle that supports your physical health and overall well-being. In doing so, you become not just a resident of the city but a thriving example of urban vitality.

In the relentless rhythm of urban life, where the cacophony of the cityscape can often overwhelm the senses, finding a sanctuary of peace within oneself becomes not just a method of coping but a vital necessity for mental and emotional well-being. Mindfulness and meditation emerge as powerful practices in this context, offering a path to tranquillity and presence in the moment, amidst the urban chaos. These practices are not just about withdrawing from the world but about engaging with it more fully, with a sense of calm and focus that enhances every aspect of one's life.

Mindfulness, the practice of being fully present and engaged in the moment, without judgment, can transform the way one experiences the city. It involves a conscious direction of our awareness to the here and now, acknowledging and accepting one's feelings, thoughts, and bodily sensations. It's about noticing the details of the world around you—the warmth of the sun on your skin, the breeze against your face, the myriad of sounds that make up the city's symphony—and finding beauty and serenity in the midst of it all.

Starting a mindfulness practice can be as simple as dedicating a few minutes each day to focus on your breathing. Sit in a quiet space, close your eyes, and take deep, slow breaths, paying attention to the sensation of air entering and leaving your body. As thoughts arise, acknowledge them without judgment and gently guide your focus back to your breath. This practice can help centre your mind, reduce stress, and enhance your sense of inner peace.

Incorporating mindfulness into daily life extends beyond dedicated sitting meditation. It can include mindful walking, where you focus fully on the experience of walking, noticing the movement of your feet, the rhythm of your breath, and the sights and sounds around you. Even routine activities like eating or washing dishes can become mindfulness practices when done with full awareness and appreciation of the moment.

Meditation, while related to mindfulness, involves specific techniques to achieve a state of deep peace and relaxation. There are various forms of meditation, including concentration meditation, where you focus on a single point of reference such as a mantra or an object; and open-monitoring meditation, where you observe all aspects of your experience, including thoughts, without attachment.

For those new to meditation, guided meditations can be a helpful starting point. Numerous apps and online resources offer guided sessions that can introduce you to the practice and help you find a style that resonates with you. Setting aside a regular time and space for meditation can help establish it as a part of your daily routine, providing a refuge of calm to return to each day.

The benefits of mindfulness and meditation are manifold, from reduced stress and anxiety to improved concentration, creativity, and emotional resilience. These practices can also enhance physical health, with research linking them to lowered blood pressure, reduced chronic pain, and improved sleep.

Furthermore, mindfulness and meditation can deepen your connections with others. By fostering a greater sense of empathy and compassion, these practices can enhance your relationships, allowing you to engage with others more fully, with kindness and understanding.

In the urban context, where the pace of life can often feel unrelenting, mindfulness and meditation offer a way to slow down, to savour each moment, and to cultivate an inner sanctuary of peace. They teach us that amidst the chaos of city life, the space for tranquillity and well-being lies within, accessible at any moment, with each breath we take.

By integrating mindfulness and meditation into your life, you can navigate the complexities of the urban environment with grace and equanimity, turning the challenges of city living into opportunities for growth and self-discovery. In doing so, you not only enhance your own well-being but also contribute to the creation of a more mindful, compassionate urban community.

In an era where the digital and physical worlds are increasingly intertwined, mastering the digital aspects of city living becomes a critical skill for anyone looking to thrive in the urban environment. The digital city offers a landscape ripe with opportunities for personal and professional growth, provided one knows how to navigate its virtual streets as adeptly as its physical ones. From harnessing the power of online networks to optimising the use of digital tools and services, the ability to leverage technology is indispensable for urban success.

The foundation of navigating the digital city lies in connectivity. Ensuring reliable access to high-speed internet is the first step, as it enables participation in the digital economy, access to information, and engagement with online communities.

In the urban context, where competition and innovation are constant, staying connected means staying informed and ahead of the curve.

Building a robust online presence is next. For professionals, platforms like LinkedIn offer a space to showcase skills, connect with industry peers, and discover job opportunities. For creatives and entrepreneurs, social media platforms can serve as a portfolio of work and a channel for marketing and engagement. Developing a clear, authentic online identity can open doors and build bridges to opportunities that might otherwise remain out of reach.

The digital city is also a hub of learning and development. Online courses, webinars, and tutorials provide access to a wealth of knowledge across every conceivable subject area. Whether it's acquiring a new skill, staying abreast of industry trends, or pursuing a personal interest, the resources available are vast and varied. Platforms like Coursera, Udemy, and Khan Academy, among others, offer courses taught by experts in their fields, making high-quality education accessible to anyone with an internet connection.

Efficiency in navigating the city's digital landscape extends to everyday tasks. Mobile apps for public transportation can simplify travel, providing real-time updates on schedules, routes, and delays. Food delivery and grocery apps bring convenience to dining and shopping, while online banking and payment services streamline financial transactions. Recognising and utilising these tools can save time, reduce stress, and enhance the quality of urban life.

The digital city also presents unique opportunities for community engagement and civic participation. Many cities have online platforms where residents can report issues, suggest improvements, and engage in dialogue with local government. Participating in these forums can foster a sense of community and empower individuals to contribute to the shaping of their urban environment.

However, navigating the digital city is not without its challenges. The issues of privacy, security, and digital well-being are paramount. Protecting personal information online requires diligence and an understanding of digital security practices, such as using strong, unique passwords and being cautious about the information shared on social media. Additionally, balancing screen time with offline activities is crucial for mental and physical health, ensuring that technology serves as a tool for enhancement rather than a source of stress.

In conclusion, the digital city offers a landscape rich with opportunities for those who know how to navigate it effectively. By building a strong online presence, leveraging digital tools for learning and efficiency, engaging with the community, and staying mindful of security and well-being, individuals can harness the power of technology for personal and professional growth. In the fast-paced urban environment, where innovation and connectivity drive progress, mastering the digital aspects of city living is not just advantageous—it's essential.

In the vibrant tapestry of city life, where the rapid pace and high demands can often lead to a sense of disconnection from one's passions and interests, finding and pursuing hobbies becomes a vital source of personal growth and enjoyment. Urban hobbies offer a unique opportunity to engage with the city's diverse offerings, carve out spaces of creativity and relaxation, and foster a deeper connection with oneself and the community. This chapter explores the myriad ways in which city dwellers can discover hobbies that not only fit into their urban lifestyle but also enrich it, providing avenues for exploration, learning, and fulfilment.

The first step in cultivating urban hobbies is to tap into the city's cultural and recreational wealth. Cities are hubs of creativity and innovation, offering a plethora of workshops, classes, and groups centred around a wide range of activities. Whether it's photography, painting, cooking, dancing, writing, or urban gardening, there's likely a community or class available. Exploring these options can spark interest in a previously unconsidered hobby or rekindle a long-lost passion. Local community centres, libraries, and online platforms are excellent resources for finding what's available. Taking the plunge and signing up for a class or workshop not only introduces you to the hobby itself but also connects you with like-minded individuals, enhancing the social aspect of your urban lifestyle.

Leveraging the urban environment itself can also inspire hobbies. Photography enthusiasts, for instance, find endless subjects in the city's architecture, street life, and changing landscapes. Urban exploration, or 'urbexing', encourages individuals to explore their city's hidden or abandoned places, offering a unique perspective on the urban environment. Running, cycling, and skateboarding can be more than just forms of exercise; they become ways to intimately know the city's streets, parks, and public spaces. The key is to see the urban environment not as a backdrop but as an active participant in your hobby.

Technology plays a significant role in cultivating hobbies in the urban context. Digital platforms and apps can introduce city dwellers to new activities and communities. From apps that guide you through historical walking tours of your city to those that connect you with local amateur sports leagues or craft circles, technology can be a gateway to discovering and deepening your engagement with urban hobbies. Furthermore, online forums and social media groups offer spaces to share experiences, seek advice, and celebrate achievements related to your hobby, thus broadening your community and support network.

Sustainability and environmental consciousness have given rise to a new category of urban hobbies. Activities like urban foraging, sustainable gardening in small spaces, and upcycling furniture not only provide personal satisfaction but also contribute positively to the environment. These hobbies encourage a deeper connection with nature and promote a sustainable lifestyle within the urban context.

Balancing hobby pursuits with the demands of urban life requires intentionality. It's about carving out time in your schedule, setting realistic goals, and prioritising activities that bring you joy and relaxation. It may involve waking up an hour earlier to write, dedicating weekend mornings to painting, or joining an evening dance class. The commitment to integrating hobbies into your life is a commitment to your well-being and happiness.

Cultivating hobbies in the city goes beyond personal enjoyment; it's about creating a balanced and enriching lifestyle amidst the hustle and bustle. Hobbies offer a counterbalance to the pressures of urban living, providing outlets for stress, opportunities for social connection, and avenues for continuous learning and creativity. They encourage us to engage with the city in new and meaningful ways, transforming the urban environment from a place of residence to a landscape of endless possibilities for growth and enjoyment. In embracing urban hobbies, we not only enrich our lives but also deepen our connection to the city and its vibrant community.

Living in a big city brings with it a kaleidoscope of experiences, opportunities, and, unavoidably, a certain level of risk. Urban environments, with their dense populations and complex socio-economic dynamics, present unique challenges to personal safety and security. However, with the right knowledge and precautions, one can navigate these risks effectively, ensuring a safe and enjoyable urban life. This chapter delves into practical advice for staying safe in a big city, covering a range of strategies from situational awareness to digital security.

Situational awareness is the cornerstone of urban safety. It involves being conscious of your environment and the people around you, understanding that situations can change rapidly. When moving through the city, whether by foot, public transport, or vehicle, keep your senses attuned to what's happening around you. This means not allowing distractions, such as smartphones or headphones, to compromise your attention. By staying alert, you can better anticipate potential dangers and react swiftly to avoid them.

The importance of familiarising yourself with your urban surroundings cannot be overstated. This means knowing the safer routes to take, the areas to avoid at certain times, and the locations of police stations and other emergency services. Make use of technology to aid in this. Map apps can provide not only directions but also information on traffic conditions, areas of high crime, and public transport updates. However, balance this reliance on technology with personal knowledge of your environment, ensuring you're not wholly dependent on digital guidance.

In terms of personal safety, adopting a few basic habits can significantly reduce risks. These include walking confidently, making eye contact with passers-by, and carrying belongings securely to deter pickpockets and thieves. When using public transport, stay in well-lit, populated areas while waiting for buses or trains, and be mindful of your possessions, especially in crowded conditions.

Nighttime in the city demands extra precautions. If you're out late, try to travel in groups, stick to well-lit, busy streets, and avoid shortcuts through isolated areas. When using taxis or ride-sharing services, verify the vehicle and driver details before getting in, and share your journey details with someone you trust.

Digital security is an aspect of urban safety that's often overlooked. In today's connected world, cyber threats are as real as physical ones. Protecting your personal information online is crucial. This includes using strong, unique passwords for different accounts, being cautious about the information you share on social media, and ensuring your devices are protected with the latest antivirus software and security updates. When accessing public Wi-Fi networks, be wary of conducting sensitive transactions, as these networks can be easily compromised.

Home security is another vital consideration. Invest in quality locks for doors and windows, and if possible, a security system or doorbell camera. Get to know your neighbours and consider joining a neighbourhood watch scheme to foster a community-based approach to safety. For apartment dwellers, securing access points and being mindful of who you let into the building can go a long way in maintaining a secure living environment.

Lastly, personal safety is not just about preventing physical harm but also about ensuring psychological well-being. The stress of constantly navigating urban risks can take a toll. Cultivate a network of friends and family you can rely on, and don't hesitate to reach out to local resources or helplines if you feel overwhelmed. Remember, the aim is not to live in fear but to equip yourself with the knowledge and skills to confidently enjoy city life.

In summary, staying safe in a big city is about combining common sense with informed precautions. By cultivating situational awareness, familiarising yourself with your environment, taking practical steps to protect yourself and your belongings, and being vigilant about digital security, you can significantly mitigate the risks associated with urban living. Embrace the vibrancy and opportunities of city life, armed with the awareness and strategies to navigate its challenges safely.

Living in the city presents a unique paradox; while it offers the allure of endless opportunities and experiences, it also poses the challenge of high living costs. However, with strategic planning and savvy decision-making, it is entirely possible to enjoy the vibrancy of urban life without compromising on financial health. This chapter explores practical tips for maximising your city budget, enabling you to savour the delights of city living affordably.

Budgeting effectively forms the bedrock of affordable urban living. It involves not just tracking your income and expenses but also setting clear priorities. Distinguish between your needs and wants, allocating funds to essential expenses like rent, utilities, and groceries before anything else. Tools and apps designed for budgeting can be incredibly helpful, offering insights into your spending patterns and helping you make informed financial decisions.

Housing, typically the largest expense in the city, requires particular attention. Consider alternative living arrangements to reduce this cost. Sharing an apartment or house with roommates can significantly cut down on rent and utilities. If you value privacy, look for smaller, less central locations where rents tend to be lower. Exploring housing options in up-and-coming neighbourhoods can also yield more affordable choices without straying too far from the city's pulse.

Transportation in the city offers multiple avenues for savings. Embrace public transit as your primary mode of getting around. Most urban centres offer comprehensive bus, tram, and train networks that are not only cost-effective but also environmentally friendly. Investing in a monthly pass can further reduce your travel expenses. For shorter distances, consider walking or cycling, which has the added benefit of promoting physical health.

Food and dining present another significant area for budget management. While the city's culinary scene is tempting, frequent dining out can quickly drain your finances. Cultivate the habit of cooking at home, relying on fresh, local produce from farmers' markets, which can be more affordable and nutritious than supermarket fare. When you do choose to eat out, look for happy hours, special deals, or choose lunch menus which are often priced more attractively than dinner menus.

Entertainment and leisure activities need not be curtailed in the pursuit of affordable urban living. Cities are rich with free or low-cost events, including outdoor concerts, museum days, public lectures, and festivals. Keep abreast of these opportunities through local newspapers, websites, or community boards. Additionally, consider volunteering as a way to participate in events or activities you enjoy; this can offer a sense of involvement and community connection without the associated costs.

Shopping smart is key to maximising your city budget. Resist the lure of impulse buys and retail therapy, focusing instead on purchasing necessities. Take advantage of sales, discount outlets, and thrift stores for clothing and other items. For furniture and home goods, online marketplaces can be a treasure trove of affordable options, especially in a city where people frequently move and sell or give away items in good condition.

Lastly, saving and investing should remain a priority, even on a tight budget. Even small amounts set aside regularly can grow over time, thanks to compound interest. Look into savings accounts with higher interest rates, or consider low-risk investments like index funds. Being financially prudent today lays the foundation for a more secure and enjoyable urban future.

In essence, affordable urban living is not about deprivation but about making thoughtful choices that align with your financial reality and life goals. By adopting a mindful approach to spending, seeking out cost-saving opportunities, and prioritising experiences over material possessions, you can fully engage with the vibrancy of city life without compromising your financial wellbeing. Embrace the challenge of budgeting as an opportunity to live more intentionally, discovering that the true essence of urban living lies not in extravagance, but in the rich tapestry of experiences the city has to offer.

In the ever-evolving landscape of the modern metropolis, the ability to adapt to urban changes and trends is not merely advantageous; it is essential for thriving in the dynamic environment of the future city. This adaptation requires a keen understanding of urban development trends, technological advancements, and the socio-economic shifts that shape our urban spaces. By preparing for these changes, individuals can not only navigate the complexities of urban living but also seize opportunities for personal and professional growth.

The future city is characterised by rapid technological innovation, shifting towards smarter, more connected urban environments. The proliferation of smart city technologies, from IoT (Internet of Things) devices to AI (Artificial Intelligence)-powered services, is transforming urban living. These technologies promise to enhance efficiency, sustainability, and quality of life, but they also require individuals to be digitally literate, able to interact with and navigate a landscape where the digital and physical increasingly merge.

Understanding and embracing these technological advancements is crucial. This means staying informed about new technologies being implemented in your city, from smart transportation systems to digital public services, and acquiring the skills necessary to use these technologies effectively. Whether it's learning to navigate app-based mobility services or understanding how to protect your privacy in an increasingly connected world, digital literacy is a key competency in the future city.

Sustainability and resilience are other critical themes in urban development. As cities face the challenges of climate change, pollution, and resource scarcity, sustainable living practices become not just ethical choices but necessities. Adapting to this trend involves adopting a sustainable lifestyle, from reducing waste and conserving energy to supporting local and sustainable businesses. It also means engaging with community efforts to make urban spaces greener and more resilient, whether through urban gardening, participation in local sustainability initiatives, or advocacy for environmental policies.

The future city also reflects significant socio-economic shifts, including changes in the job market, housing trends, and community dynamics. The rise of the gig economy, remote work, and co-living spaces are examples of trends that are reshaping how we work and live. Adapting to these changes requires flexibility and a willingness to explore new modes of working and living. It might mean considering alternative career paths, embracing remote work opportunities, or exploring new forms of housing that offer both affordability and community.

Community engagement and social inclusion are becoming increasingly important in urban development. The future city is not just a space of technological and economic activity but a community where diversity is celebrated, and social cohesion is strengthened. Engaging with your community, whether through local events, civic initiatives, or volunteerism, can enrich your urban experience and ensure you are an active participant in shaping the future of your city.

Finally, preparing for the future city involves a commitment to lifelong learning. The pace of change in urban environments means that the skills and knowledge that are relevant today may evolve tomorrow. Staying curious, seeking out learning opportunities, and being open to new experiences are essential for keeping pace with the changes and ensuring that you remain adaptable and resilient in the face of urban transformations.

In summary, adapting to urban changes and trends requires a multifaceted approach. It involves embracing technological advancements, adopting sustainable practices, navigating socio-economic shifts, engaging with your community, and committing to continuous learning. By understanding and preparing for these developments, individuals can not only survive but thrive in the future city, seizing opportunities for innovation, growth, and connection in an ever-changing urban landscape.

Embarking on a journey of self-discovery and personal development through self-assessment requires courage, honesty, and a willingness to face one's true self. It is a profound process that not only unveils your inherent strengths but also exposes vulnerabilities and areas needing improvement. This exploration is essential for anyone aspiring to thrive in the complexities of modern life, allowing for a tailored approach to personal growth and professional advancement.

The initial step in this introspective journey involves reflecting on past experiences, both successes and failures, to identify patterns in your behaviour and decision-making. Such reflection can illuminate your natural inclinations and abilities, highlighting strengths that have consistently contributed to your achievements. Equally, it can reveal weaknesses or gaps in your skillset that may have hindered progress or led to setbacks. Keeping a reflective journal can facilitate this process, offering a structured way to document and analyse these insights over time.

Feedback from peers, colleagues, and mentors is another invaluable resource in the self-assessment process. Often, others can provide perspective on our abilities and behaviours that we might overlook or underestimate. Seeking constructive feedback, therefore, is not a sign of weakness but a demonstration of openness to growth and learning. However, it is crucial to approach this feedback with discernment, distinguishing between helpful insights and comments that may not reflect your true capabilities or intentions.

Personality assessments and skill inventories can offer a more structured approach to self-assessment. Tools such as the Myers-Briggs Type Indicator (MBTI) or the StrengthsFinder assessment provide frameworks for understanding your personality traits, working styles, and innate strengths. While these tools should not be seen as definitive labels, they can serve as useful starting points for deeper self-exploration and development planning.

Setting specific, measurable, achievable, relevant, and time-bound (SMART) goals is a critical next step in applying the insights gained from self-assessment. These goals should address both leveraging your strengths and addressing your weaknesses, with a clear plan for action. For instance, if a key strength is effective communication, you might set a goal to enhance this skill further by leading workshops or presentations. Conversely, if a notable weakness is time management, a goal might involve adopting new strategies or tools to improve productivity and efficiency.

Continuous learning and development are central to this journey. The landscape of skills and competencies required for success is ever-evolving, necessitating a commitment to lifelong learning. This could involve formal education, such as courses or workshops, or more informal methods, such as reading, mentorship, or practice. The aim is to maintain a growth mindset, viewing each challenge as an opportunity to learn and each failure as a lesson.

In conclusion, self-assessment is not a one-time task but a continuous process of reflection, feedback, and goal setting. It demands honesty, resilience, and a proactive approach to personal and professional development. By regularly evaluating your strengths and weaknesses, seeking constructive feedback, and committing to targeted goals and continuous learning, you can navigate the path of self-improvement with confidence and clarity. This process not only enhances your current abilities but also prepares you for the challenges and opportunities of the future, enabling you to lead a fulfilling and successful life.

Urban Symphony
In the city's heart beats a vibrant drum,
A symphony of sounds, where dreams come from.
Skyscrapers reach, touching the sky,
Underneath, the city's pulse throbs high.
Taxi horns blare in a rhythmic dance,
Neon lights flicker, giving romance.
Footsteps echo on rain-slick streets,
In every alley, adventure meets.
A mosaic of faces, stories untold,
In the bustling market, fortunes are sold.
The city breathes, alive and fierce,
In every corner, the world it pierces.

Midnight in the Metropolis

Midnight cloaks the city's sprawl,
Silent whispers, a distant call.
The moonlight bathes the streets in glow,
Unveiling secrets only night will know.
Empty cafes, deserted parks,
Beneath the bridge, the water marks.
A cat prowls, a lone car speeds,
The city's heart at night still beats.
Stars peek through the urban haze,
A rare sight, on clear nights, a gaze.
In the quiet, the city finds its peace,
A brief respite, a soft release.

Concrete Jungle
In the jungle of concrete and steel,
Survival requires an iron will.
Rivers of people flow down the street,
In the urban wild, strangers meet.
Graffiti blooms on a subway car,
A spray-painted, neon-lit star.
Parks nestled between towers tall,
Green oases, free for all.
The city roars, a living beast,
On energy and dreams, it feasts.
Yet in its heart, beauty resides,
In moments of calm, it confides.

City of Dreams

A city of dreams, where tales unfold,
In whispered tones, bold and bold.
Each street corner tells a story,
Of struggle, triumph, and fleeting glory.
Lights shimmer, a beacon for seekers,
Artists, workers, and midnight speakers.
Every face in the crowd, a dream alight,
Chasing visions in the fading light.
Skyscrapers stand as sentinels tall,
Witness to rise, and witness to fall.
In the city's embrace, we find our place,
In its boundless grace, a relentless chase.

Moving to a big city is an adventure filled with excitement, opportunities, and challenges. Whether you're relocating for a job, education, or for the sheer experience of urban life, navigating the complexities of a metropolis requires preparation and adaptability. This guide outlines essential steps to help you transition smoothly into your new urban environment.

1. Research and Plan Ahead
- **Choose the Right Neighbourhood:** Consider factors like safety, proximity to work or school, access to public transportation, and the availability of amenities. Online forums, city guides, and local news websites can offer valuable insights.
- **Understand the Cost of Living:** Big cities often come with higher living expenses. Research the cost of rent,

food, transportation, and utilities to create a realistic budget.

2. Secure Accommodation
- **Start Your Search Early:** Competition for housing in big cities can be fierce. Use online property listings, real estate agents, and social networks to find suitable options.
- **Consider Temporary Housing:** If you're unable to secure long-term accommodation before moving, short-term rentals or serviced apartments can provide a base while you continue your search.

3. Manage Logistics
- **Hire a Reliable Moving Company:** Look for movers with experience in urban relocations. They can navigate challenges like narrow streets and apartment building restrictions.
- **Downsize Your Belongings:**

Space is at a premium in city apartments. Sell, donate, or store items you don't need to make your move easier and your new home less cluttered.

4. Get to Know the Public Transport System
- **Familiarise Yourself with Routes and Schedules:** Big cities boast extensive public transport networks. Understanding how to navigate buses, trains, and subways will make your life much easier.
- **Invest in a Transit Pass:** Many cities offer travel cards or passes that provide cost-effective and convenient access to public transport.

5. Build a New Network
- **Join Local Groups and Clubs:** Engage with communities that share your interests or hobbies. This is a

great way to meet people and make friends.
- **Utilise Social Media and Apps:** Platforms like Meetup and local Facebook groups can connect you with events and social gatherings in your area.

6. Stay Safe and Secure
- **Learn About Local Safety:** Educate yourself on the city's safer areas and those to avoid, especially at night. Always be aware of your surroundings.
- **Update Your Address:** Ensure your address is up-to-date with banks, government agencies, and other important institutions for your security and to receive mail.

7. Embrace the Lifestyle
- **Explore Your Surroundings:** Spend your first few weeks visiting

local landmarks, parks, museums, and restaurants to get a feel for the city's culture.
- **Be Open to New Experiences:** Big cities are melting pots of diversity and opportunity. Say yes to new experiences, whether it's trying different cuisines, attending cultural events, or exploring new neighbourhoods.

8. Take Care of Your Well-being
- **Find Your Quiet Places:** Discover parks or cafes where you can unwind and escape the hustle and bustle when needed.
- **Maintain a Healthy Lifestyle:** Seek out local gyms, fitness classes, or outdoor activities to keep physically active amidst the urban rush.

9. Stay Financially Savvy
- **Track Your Spending:** Living in a

big city can be expensive, especially when you're soaking up new experiences. Keep an eye on your finances to avoid overspending.
- **Look for Deals and Discounts:** Take advantage of happy hours, discount days at museums, and city discount cards to enjoy what the city has to offer without breaking the bank.

10. Be Patient and Give Yourself Time to Adjust
- **Expect a Period of Adjustment:** It takes time to acclimate to the pace and lifestyle of a big city. Be patient with yourself as you navigate the initial challenges and homesickness.

Moving to a big city is a transformative experience that promises growth, adventure, and countless stories. By planning ahead, staying informed, and embracing the journey with an open mind and heart, you'll pave the way for a fulfilling urban life.

The Allure of Urban Life: Why Moving to a Big City Might Be Your Best Decision Yet

The prospect of moving to a big city can be as daunting as it is exciting. The hustle and bustle, the sea of unfamiliar faces, and the seemingly endless maze of streets offer a stark contrast to the tranquility and familiarity of smaller towns or rural areas. Yet, every year, millions are drawn to these urban behemoths, seeking what they cannot find elsewhere. The allure of big city living is not without reason; it's rooted in a myriad of opportunities for personal and professional growth, cultural enrichment, and a lifestyle that's as dynamic as the cityscape itself. Here are compelling reasons why moving to a big city might just be the leap worth taking.

Unparalleled Career Opportunities

Big cities are often the engines of the economy, home to multinational corporations, booming industries, and startups in cutting-edge sectors. This concentration of businesses provides a wealth of employment opportunities across a spectrum of fields, offering not just jobs but careers that can propel individuals to new heights of professional achievement. Whether you're an aspiring artist, a tech enthusiast, or a finance professional, urban centers offer the fertile ground necessary for planting the seeds of a successful career.

Cultural Melting Pot

One of the most enriching aspects of big city life is its diversity. Cities are melting pots of cultures, bringing together people from various backgrounds, ethnicities, and walks of life. This cultural amalgamation fosters an environment of learning and exchange, where one can indulge in international cuisines, participate in cultural festivals, and interact with people from different perspectives, enriching one's worldview and fostering a sense of global citizenship.

Endless Entertainment and Leisure Activities

Boredom is a word seldom uttered by city dwellers. With an array of museums, theaters, galleries, and clubs, the city's cultural and entertainment offerings are virtually limitless. Whether it's catching a Broadway show, visiting an art exhibit, enjoying a live music performance, or exploring the latest culinary trends, big cities provide an endless array of activities to fill your leisure time and enrich your life outside work.

Educational Institutions and Resources

For those keen on furthering their education, big cities offer unparalleled access to prestigious universities, research institutions, and libraries. The concentration of academic resources, coupled with the opportunity to attend lectures, workshops, and seminars by leading experts, makes cities ideal for students and lifelong learners alike. Moreover, the networking opportunities available can be instrumental in building a solid foundation for one's future career.

Networking and Personal Growth

The sheer number of people living in big cities increases the likelihood of meeting like-minded individuals, industry leaders, and potential mentors who can play a significant role in your personal and professional development. Networking events, conferences, and social gatherings are more plentiful and varied, providing ample opportunities to connect with others and forge relationships that can lead to new ventures, collaborations, or career advancements.

Public Transportation and Connectivity

While traffic congestion might be a downside, the extensive public transportation networks in big cities—from subways and buses to bikeshares—make getting around more accessible and environmentally friendly than in car-dependent locales. This connectivity not only facilitates daily commutes but also encourages exploration of the city's diverse neighborhoods and attractions.

A Test of Independence and Resilience

Living in a big city can be a profound personal test, challenging one's ability to adapt, overcome obstacles, and navigate the complexities of urban life. The experience fosters independence, resilience, and a can-do attitude that can serve individuals well in all areas of life. It's a place where you learn to trust in your abilities and push beyond your comfort zone.

Embracing the Urban Adventure

Moving to a big city is not merely a

change of address; it's a leap into a vast world of opportunities, experiences, and personal growth. The challenges of urban living are real, but the rewards—professional advancement, cultural enrichment, and the sheer thrill of being part of the vibrant tapestry of city life—are immeasurable. If you're contemplating this move, you might just find that the big city holds the keys to unlocking your potential and transforming your dreams into reality.